LOW CALORIES

Foods to Eat to Lose Weight and Stay Healthy.
Includes 1,200 to 1,700-Calorie Meal Plans

Nancy Peterson

Copyright @ 2019

TABLE OF CONTENT

Introduction 4

What is the Low-Calorie Diet? 5

Background of the Low-Calorie Diet 7

How Does the Diet Works? 8

Extreme Low-Calorie Diets 9

Dangers of Extreme Low-Calorie Diets 9

Reasons to Try the Low-Calorie Diet 10

What Happens When You Restrict Calories? 11

Who Should Go on Low-Calorie Diet? 14

What are Low-Calorie Foods 15

How to Start the Low Calories Diet 17

How to Follow a Low-Calorie Diet 18

How Soon Do You See Results? 19

How Many Calories a Day Should I Eat 19

How Does the Weight Loss Calculator Work? 20

How to Use the Weight Loss Calculator 21

How to Count Your Daily Calories Intake 23

Tips on Effective Calorie Counts 24

Tips and Resources to Succeed 27

USDA Recommendations 29

Pros and Cons of the Low-Calories Diet 29

Foods to Eat 33

Foods to Reduce 34

1,200-Calorie Diet Meal Plan 36

1,500-Calorie Diet Meal Plan 40

1,700-Calorie Diet Meal Plan 46

Reaching Your Weight Loss Goal 50

Explaining High-Intensity Interval Training (HIIT), ... 53

Weight Training 58

Recommendations for Weight Training 59

Intermittent Fasting 61

How Effective is Intermittent Fasting for Weight Loss?. 62

Conclusion 63

Other Books by Nancy Peterson 64

Introduction

If you have tried the low-calorie diet in the past, you may not fancy the idea of cutting calories every day. However, most of the diets that exist require that you reduce your calorie intake in one way or the other. Some diets would require that you consume foods that contain fewer calories but fills up faster like vegetables and fruits in place of processed foods. While some other diets restrict your options making you eat the same thing over and again which becomes less interesting as time goes on. The remaining diets have a mix of both strategies, like making a special shake for most of your meals or recommending low-calorie foods like tomatoes. Now, new research has proven that being on a low-calorie diet would help you to lose excess weight faster than other diets. In this book, you would learn everything there is to know about the low-calorie diet including what it is all about, foods to eat when embarking on a low-calorie diet, foods to avoid, tips to succeed in this diet as well as sample meal plans to guide you in achieving great results with this diet. This book has been written in a simple language to ensure that everyone who picks this book understands the content of the book and is able to have a fun and interesting time while counting calories and dropping that excess weight.

What is the Low-Calorie Diet?

This is a diet that restricts your calorie intake to 1,000 to 1,200 calories daily for women and 1,200 to 1,700 calories daily for men. Some people tend to go on a very low-calorie diet to achieve a swift weight loss which involves consuming only 800 calories daily. This type of diet has more special foods like bars, shakes or soups in place of meals. While you can lose up to 3 to 5 pounds of weight every week with a very low-calorie diet, it is not advisable except if instructed by your medical doctor or nutritionist. If your aim is to lose weight, you should go for a low-calorie diet against the very low-calorie diet. It is easier to follow diets that are not too extreme as they do not interrupt your daily activities as much as other diets and are also less risky for persons with other health problems or over 50 years. Also, some people who go on a very low-calorie diet have complained of gallstones. It is important to remember that for this diet to work, you also have to make healthy lifestyle choices which include reducing your sedentary time per day and increasing your daily exercises. When you follow the low-calorie diet, it creates a calorie deficit in the body which in turn leads to weight loss. The diet is known to be very effective but would take discipline for it to work as well as be safe.

Again, like I always mention in my diet books, it is very important that you consult your doctor before you begin this diet so that you do not restrict your calories more than is necessary as well as not lose out on nutrients that your body needs for its day to day functions. According to Chrissy Carroll, RD, MPH, this diet is not for breastfeeding women and athletes.

Background of the Low-Calorie Diet

Several types of research have been carried out on this diet from as far back as the 1980s to verify claims that the diet can help to slow down the aging process. The science behind weight loss is simple: consume fewer calories than your body needs (via deliberate exercise and daily living) and you lose weight ultimately. However, do not assume that because the science is simple means that the diet is also too simple to follow. You would need to plan well and put in much effort to overcome the hunger signs and ensure that the 1,000 to 1,500 calories that you consume daily supplies your body with all the fuel and the right nutrients that the body needs. This is the main reason breastfeeding and pregnant women are advised not to go for this diet as they would need enough calories for themselves and their babies. Athletes are also advised not to go on this diet as they need sufficient calories to provide energy for them to perform.

How Does the Diet Works?

Before you decide to start the low-calorie diet, I would advise that you go for a physical examination. This is more important for persons that have health conditions like high cholesterol or high blood pressure. Measure your body composition and then set your goals. For instance, you can take measurement of your body mass index (BMI) as well as your waist circumference, which are two measures asides your weight that can help to show your weight loss progress. Once this is done, the next step would be to know how many calories per day your body needs. This step differs from one person to another and tends to change as time goes on. You need to determine how many calories you need per day to sustain your current weight, then deduct the figure by 100 to 500 calories. When starting, it is advisable that you begin with a small calorie reduction as it may become difficult to sustain if you go all in from the start.

Extreme Low-Calorie Diets

This type of diet involves eating foods that contain less than 800 calories per day. While some people would want to undergo an extremely low-calorie diet as a faster way to lose weight, it is very important that it is done only under a doctor's supervision. The Extreme low-calorie diet has to do with consuming low-calorie shakes, supplements or meal replacements. You also need to carry out frequent blood tests to measure things like blood lipids, micronutrients, electrolyte levels, white and red blood cell count, blood pressure and blood sugar levels. These tests are very important if you decide to go for the extreme low-calorie diet as the diet does not give the body all the nutrition that the body needs and this can negatively affect the factors mentioned above and in turn, harm your health.

Dangers of Extreme Low-Calorie Diets

This type of diet may work if you need to lose weight in a very short time but they are also very risky to your health as they do not give the body sufficient nutrients and calories that the body needs to function optimally. For most people, it is advisable to stay at a minimum of 1,200 calories daily. The diet is not sustainable and you may end up gaining more weight as soon as you are done with the diet. According to Lindsay Malone who is a clinical dietician at Cleveland Clinic, people who go on the extreme low diet and not getting sufficient protein are pushing their body to risk as the body tends to dip into the muscle stores for energy.

Reasons to Try the Low-Calorie Diet

The major reason to go on the low-calorie diet is for weight loss. What other good reasons are there to give up on foods that you love. However, research on animal studies showed more benefits of calorie reduction. According to the review in *Molecular Aspects of Medicine* in June 2011, research shows that animals including primates that were subjected to calorie restriction experienced the following:

- Higher levels of physical activity
- Longer lives
- Improved reproductive performance
- Reduced age-related brain degeneration
- Reduced rate of cancer

Some parts of this finding may seem somewhat odd to persons who have tried to either fast or restrict their calorie intake and then experienced early fatigue, nausea, lack of energy, weakness and stomach pains from their efforts. However, these animal studies and observations included regular periods of restricting calories backed up with a healthy diet. What this means is that the bodies of these animals had sufficient time to adapt to the less caloric intake in a healthy manner over a long period of time.

What Happens When You Restrict Calories?

Most times when people talk about cutting down their calorie intake for heart health, they do not talk about doing it to feel better, live longer and enjoy an improved quality of life. This is mostly because we look at the short-term goal and how it would make us feel in the first few days or weeks after starting rather than looking at it on a long-term outlook.

One study published in June 2016 in *JAMA Internal Medicine* gave a unique insight into what happens to the human body when we restrict our calorie intake. The study included participants that were not obese especially because obese people need to lose weight in order to reduce the risk of having sleep apnea, high blood pressure, diabetes, and coronary artery disease as well as to improve their quality of life. The researchers studied 218 participants for two years. 70 percent of the participants were women while the average age of participants was 38. To qualify for enrollment, the body mass index (BMI) of participants could be up to 28 but not less than 22. The participants were divided into two groups, one group on the low-calorie diet and the other group were asked to continue with their normal diet. Those on a restricted-calorie diet consumed approximately 25% fewer calories than their usual intake. You may be wondering why the researchers went for a 25% reduction in calories. They considered it the safest and lowest level that can be sustained for the whole 2 years period of the study. Participants met in their groups and also were given web-based resources that helped them with their diet. Registered dietitians were also engaged to monitor the weekly food diaries of participants to be able to determine their total calories. Every one of the participants was advised to exercise for a minimum of 5 days a week, 30 minutes at a time.

The researchers reported their findings at the end of the research. The first which is not surprising is that participants that consumed lesser calories lost more weight. Participants in this group, on average, lost 16.7 lbs. (7.6 kg) compared to participants in the second group that lost 0.9 lbs. (0.4 kg).

The best part of the finding was the impact the restriction on calories had on the quality of life of participants. Participants on restricted calories reported that they experienced less daily tension, better moods, and they also confirmed to have felt better all through the study. The group placed on calorie restriction also confirmed that they experienced quality and longer sleep, more sexual drive, and arousal as well as better sexual relationships than participants from the other group.

Who Should Go on Low-Calorie Diet?

For persons that are obese or overweight, it's quite a simple choice to make. It is important to lose excess weight for your general health as well as to reduce your chances of premature joint disease, cancer, diabetes, cardiovascular disease, high blood pressure, and sleep apnea. But these are not all the benefits that come from reducing your calorie intake. Several other benefits of this diet can help to improve the quality of your life and your daily functioning.

For those within the normal weight range, studies suggest that there are potential benefits if you carefully follow the diet and ensure that your BMI does not go below 22. If you decide to cut down on your calorie intake, it is important to follow the suggestion of the researchers in this study and carry out only a 25% reduction. This is the level that your body can tolerate while still benefiting from the diet.

What are Low-Calorie Foods

We have different versions of this low-calorie diet. One example worthy of note is a Professor of human nutrition at Kansas State University, who in 2010, dropped 27 pounds within two months by sticking to snack chips, Twinkies and sugary cereals. The professor restricted himself to consume foods with less than 1,800 calories each day which he called the "convenience store diet." Although we have several low calories diets, all of them promote eating meals that are high in nutrients and low in calories. According to a registered dietician with Pritikin Longevity Center in Miami, Goscilo and Kimberly Gomer, the foods below are foods that make up a low-calorie diet:

Breakfast

- Tea or coffee – 1 cup
- Oatmeal with any fresh fruit of choice and no added sugar.

Lunch

- Fresh fruit, like Apple or Pear – 1 piece /carrots – ½ cup
- Water
- Sliced deli turkey breast with whole-grain bread – 2 slices

Dinner

- Steamed asparagus, broccoli or other vegetables – 1 cup
- Broiled or baked flounder or salmon – 3-ounce piece
- Fat-free pudding – 1 cup

Snacks

- Yogurt with fresh fruit
- Edamame
- Air-popped popcorn

- High-fiber crackers with low-fat cheese
- Apples
- Veggies with hummus

How to Start the Low Calories Diet

The points below are a summary of what you need to know to be successful with the low-calorie diet.

- Keep an accurate record of your food consumption for about one to 2 weeks
- Make use of online calorie counters to know your daily calorie intake.
- Make plans to reduce your intake of calories by 25% by the next month.
- Draw out a menu plan each week that has all your favorites food in it.

One best and easy way to reduce calories is by increasing the number of vegetables and whole fruits that you consume which would help to fill you quickly and contains fewer calories. Also, you can make the diet change with other people be it friends or family that can render social support and accountability. This is a powerful factor that can improve the chances of your success on this diet. As soon as you start to experience improved sleep, quality of life and other benefits, it would help to positively push you to continue on your goal and make a daily habit of restricting calories. As you become better, you would notice that your visit to the local cardiologist would reduce.

How to Follow a Low-Calorie Diet

It is advised that you follow this diet under the supervision of your physician and/ or a registered dietician. It is important that you always get enough nutrients while on this diet and this can only be achieved with the help of dietetic and medical professionals. You can also make use of free apps like **MyFitnessPal,** to record your daily food intake. Apps like this help you to keep track of the number of calories that you burn daily each time you record your activities.

How Soon Do You See Results?

The low-calorie diet does not take a long time before yielding results. The number of calories that you take as well as your level of activity plays an important role when it comes to achieving results on this diet. But be rest assured that this diet can guarantee you losing some pounds within the first few weeks of starting the diet.

How Many Calories a Day Should I Eat

Some calorie calculators are very useful in calculating how many calories you should eat daily to maintain your weight. Some even go as far as telling you what you need to gain weight. But our purpose here is to lose weight and for this, you would need a weight loss calculator. One that can tell you how many calories you should consume daily to hit your weight loss mark. It is quite a simple process to calculate the number of calories needed for weight loss, weight maintenance or weight gain. All you need to do is follow the steps I have highlighted below and you would be able to tell what you need to achieve your goal.

How Does the Weight Loss Calculator Work?

This calculator has a very simple procedure that can even be fun and interesting while working towards your goal. You may be wondering how a calorie counter works. When you input data in the calculator, it makes use of a formula known as the **Mifflin St. Jeor equation** to get your resting metabolic rate. This rate tells the number of calories that your body would need for it to function when the body is at rest. Then the calculator makes use of the personalized lifestyle information that you have inputted and adds the calories that are needed to fuel your body for its daily activity. It then either subtracts calories to achieve weight loss or adds calories to achieve weight gain. If you have lost the needed pounds and just want to maintain your current weight, the calculator can tell you how much calories you need to consume to maintain the current weight. This is beneficial for people who are healthy eaters. If you have a healthy weight and would want to maintain your body size, it is important that you do not eat too little or too much. For some adults, this means sticking to a diet of 2,000 calories. However, we are all different in sizes, some are more active while some are less active and we all have different calorie needs.

How to Use the Weight Loss Calculator

Before you can get any result from the calculator, you need to first input basic information like your gender, age, current weight, and height, to get the correct number of calories. The calculator needs this data as they are important factors that can influence your metabolic rate/ the calories that you need to consume for your body to function properly. Generally, men are to consume more calories than the female gender. Bigger bodies require more calories than persons with smaller bodies while young adults need more calories than seniors. You would also need to provide your activity habits. If you are more active during the day, the body would require additional fuel (more calories). It is advisable that you are as sincere as possible when inputting your exercise habits as well as daily activities. If you do not put in the correct numbers, you would not get the correct result. If you are not particularly sure of your activeness during the day, you can have a journal handy where you record your activity for one week or even make use of your fitness tracker to get an estimate of your activity level.

After you have inputted your activity level, the next would be to input your goals/ desire. You need to be realistic at this point. Try to set a goal that you can achieve so that you do not get discouraged early. For example, if you want to go down to 130 pounds and you know that for the most part of your life you have never gone below 160 pounds, it may not be realistic at the time to assume a goal of 130. However, you can always set new goals as soon as you achieve the current goals.

The final step would be to choose a date when you would want the goal to be achieved. For persons trying to lose weight, 0.5 to 2 pounds of weight loss each week is considered a healthy rate. For persons trying to gain weight, you may succeed in gaining up to 1 pound every week.

How to Count Your Daily Calories Intake

To be able to achieve your weight loss goals, you need to learn how to correctly count your calories intake. You have more than one way you can monitor your daily calorie intake as we have already established. You can make use of websites like LoseIt or MyFitnessPal or download similar apps on your smartphone. These services would require you to input the meals that you consumed as well as the portion size after which it would automatically calculate how many calories you had in a day. You also have activity trackers like the Fitbit, that helps you to keep a record of your daily exercises and food calories. If you do not fancy tech gadgets, you can make use of a paper food journal to write down all your calorie intake or simply use a daily food intake sheet to record your numbers.

Tips on Effective Calorie Counts

- You need a portable calorie-tracking device. It may be more effective to first record the calories in your meal before you consume the meal. This is why you should have a portable tracker that you can take anywhere. This could either be a small notebook or even an app on your mobile device.
- Do not totally rely on your memory. You may not always be able to tell all that you ate in a day even if you are not on a diet. Even if you remember what you ate today, it is almost impossible to be able to tell the number of calories you consumed correctly. This is why it is important to record your activities daily.
- Don't determine portion sizes by guesswork. It is normal for humans to underestimate our food portions. We all have that particular food that we tend to overeat. An example is a cereal. Most people just keep refilling their bowl with

cereals without knowing the exact portion sizes.
- Get a kitchen scale. If you want to correctly tell how much calories are in a meal, then you should get a kitchen scale. The scale would be able to tell you the exact serving size of a meal. You do not need to use the scale each time you want to eat but you can use it when eating new food. Weigh some part of the food so that you can know how much to eat. Knowing how many grams are in a serving would help you to get the right calorie count.
- Let it be a habit to write down everything. As long as it is going into your mouth, you need to write it down. You may end up surprised knowing how these foods we call small end up adding a big number to your weight loss results.
- Always record your nibbles or snacks. Snacks or nibbles should not be left out of the record. Every few bites you take from a partner's dessert counts.

- You do not need expensive tools to achieve results. That they are expensive does not mean they are the most effective. The best calorie tracking tool is the one that works for you regardless of the price.
- Only go for tools that are fit for your lifestyle. If you spend most of your time in front of a computer, the online tool may be perfect for you. For some others, the diet app on their mobile device is the best choice for them. While for some other people, they achieve better results by using the traditional pen and paper.
- Don't be limited to tracking calories alone. To reach your weight loss target, the total number of calories you take every day is very important. For example, dieters that need to gain lean muscle mass would also need to eat the right amount of protein. And depending on the tools you are using; you can track things like your sodium and calcium intake. You can also use the app to confirm that you have the right amount of exercise for your weight loss goal.

- Also, ensure to record the major nutrients. While recording your total calories, you need to also record the carbohydrate, protein and fat grams contained in the foods that you eat. Another good number that you should not miss out include fiber and trans-fat content. When you increase your fiber intake and eliminate trans-fat from your diet, it would help to improve your health.

Tips and Resources to Succeed

To be able to count calories, you should be able to tell how much food you consume per meal. You can use a kitchen scale with some measuring cups to measure out all your servings until you are able to comfortably estimate your portions visually. Don't forget that your beverages may also contain calories and so there is a need to measure your liquid intake. For increased chances of success in this diet, you need to keep a record of all the foods you consume. Have a notebook where you record your food intake or make use of apps like MyFitnessPal or the ones that come with fitness gadgets like Apple Watch or Fitbit. You can also make use of online diet sites to keep a record of your food intake as well as grade your daily diet for its nutritional value. Keeping a food diary would also help you to see habits that are not allowing you to progress with your weight loss goals like when you consume food as a reward or for comfort.

Additional Tips

- Pack your lunch before going to school or work to give you better control over what you eat and to help reduce the temptation of indulging in junk food or fast food.
- Rather than high-calorie beverages, consume more water, lots of it.
- When eating out, always go for salad or vegetable soups. Be careful with the dressings and other toppings that are high in calories.
- The more physical exercise and activities you do, the more calories you burn.

USDA Recommendations

The USDA, as a general rule, suggests that 2000 calories per day be used for weight maintenance while 1900 and below calories per day should be used for weight loss. The low-calories diet goes further by reducing the calorie intake to 1500 and below. However, the diet supports a balanced nutritional intake that goes in line with the USDA guideline. For more information on the USDA recommendations, please visit the website https://www.choosemyplate.gov/

Pros and Cons of the Low-Calories Diet

Pros

- The diet is safe to practice
- It is very effective
- Foods for this diet are easily accessible

Now, let me explain each of the points that we have mentioned.

Effectiveness

If you follow the diet carefully, you would notice that it is quite effective especially when it is done on a short-term basis. To maintain the weight loss, you would need to further reduce your calorie intake from what it was during the weight loss time. Each time you lose weight, it also reduces your body's calorie requirement and so, you would need to adjust your calorie intake. Let's not forget that the main goal of this diet is to maintain good health.

Accessibility

The low-calorie diet is not asking you to go for specialty foods or supplements. All you need are the regular, real foods that you see in your neighborhood supermarket, although you may need to go for the low-fat or low-calorie version of foods like dairy products.

Safety

This diet is considered safe as long as it is done under medical supervision and advises. With the help of a nutritionist or doctor, you would be guided on what to eat to get sufficient nutrients and calories that your body needs to stay safe and healthy. The safety and effectiveness of the diet are dependent on how you follow the guidelines as advised by your nutritionist or doctor.

Cons

- May lead to increased appetite
- Not for everyone
- Requires tracking and careful planning

Hunger

Whenever you consume lesser calories than your body is used to, you would definitely get hungry in no time. This diet can cause weight gain when stopped, however, you can help by eating slowly and ensuring to thoroughly chew your foods mouthful by mouthful.

Also, always drink lots of water. Your body always needs the fluids and you do not have to worry as water has no calories in it. For additional flavor, you can add lemon or lime slices to the water.

Practicality

To be successful with the low-calorie diet, you have to involve lots of planning and careful tracking of your calorie intake. Unlike the extreme calorie diet that involves meal replacements only, the low-calorie diet would require you to make your own decisions. You are in complete charge of your food intake, what you eat, when you eat and how much you eat.

Appropriateness

Like was said earlier in this book, the diet is not for everyone. It is always important you get a go-ahead from your doctor before starting any weight loss diet plan. Breastfeeding and pregnant women, in particular, should avoid this diet.

Foods to Eat

- Herbs and spices
- Lean proteins
- Whole grains
- Vegetables
- Fruits
- Low or no-fat dairy products

Because you are reducing the number of calories that you consume, it is important that you ensure that every calorie that goes into your body counts. This is why you need to go for only foods that have a high nutrient quantity. Foods that are rich in fiber would also help to make you feel full.

Fruits and Vegetables

These are the perfect choice for the low-calorie diet as they offer you less of what you do not want which is the fat and calories while supplying you with more of what your body needs; fiber and nutrients.

Low-Fat Dairy and Lean Proteins

Sources of lean protein include grilled fish, chicken, and low-fat dairy products. They remove the extra calories in fat and still give you the protein that your body needs.

Whole Grains

You cannot totally make away with carbohydrates as your body needs them. But you have to go for the right one which is the whole grains that would supply more nutrients to your body along with your calories.

Herbs and Spices

These add flavor to your food without adding calories and fat. However, it is important that you watch your intake of sodium.

Foods to Reduce

- Sweetened beverages
- Rich, fatty foods (excess intake)
- Refined carbohydrates (excess intake)

Rich, Fatty Foods (in Excess)

While it is not advisable to totally leave out these foods from your menu, you would need to ensure that they do not make up most of your daily calorie intake as you may end up regretting the decision. These foods include butter, fatty cuts of meat, oil, cheese, and sugar. They contain lots of calories and would fill up your required calorie intake faster without achieving the desired results. This also applies to sweetened beverages. You can make use of non-nutritive or artificial sweeteners to reduce your calorie intake but it is better that you concentrate more on good foods rather than sugar-free junk foods. That said, you can still treat yourself to 100 to 150 calories daily be it chips, candies, or any other sweet treat. Just be conscious of the portions so that you do not eat more than you should. You can also go for healthier treats like a small glass of red wine or dark chocolate rather than purely junk foods. The antioxidants contained in the 2 examples may be good for your body.

Refined Carbohydrates (in Excess)

There are no foods that you should totally remove from your diet in the low-calorie diet. But it is important not to fill up your daily calorie quantity from simple carbs while missing out on important nutrients. These carbs would also make you feel hungry faster.

1,200-Calorie Diet Meal Plan

To start your menu plan, you would need to select foods that are low in calories and high in fiber like vegetables and fruits, low-fat protein sources and whole grains. Below, I have included two 1,200 calories daily menu to help you get started. The first is a 1,215-calorie menu that does not have any non-nutritive sweeteners added to it.

Breakfast

- Oatmeal – 1 cup
- Honey – 1 tablespoon
- Non-fat milk – ½ cup
- Plain tea or coffee as a beverage – 1 cup

- Blueberries – ½ cup

Lunch

- Water as a beverage
- 100% whole grain bread – 2 slices, tomato slice, deli-sliced turkey breast, mustard, and lettuce – 1 tablespoon
- Sliced carrots – ½ cup

Dinner

- Water with a slice of lemon
- Green beans – 1 cup
- Baked salmon – 3-ounces
- Salad with raw spinach – 1 cup, broccoli florets – ½ cup and cherry tomatoes - 5. Use lemon juice for dressing

Snacks

- Strawberries – 1 cup
- Several cups of water
- One apple with 12 almonds

- Plain yogurt - ½ cup with honey – 1 tablespoon
- Non-fat milk – 1 cup

Nutritional Information

- **Total calories:** 1,215
- **Fiber:** 28 grams
- **Total Fat:** 17.7%

- **Total Carbohydrates:** 59.3%
- **Total Protein:** 23%
- **Sodium:** 1,402 milligrams
- **Cholesterol:** 94 milligrams
- **Sugar:** 107 grams
- **Saturated Fat:** 5 grams

This second meal plan is a 1,218-calorie menu that does not have any non-nutritive sweeteners added to it.

Breakfast

- Whole-grain corn cereal – 1 cup
- Non-fat milk – ½ cup
- Sucralose – 1 packet

- 100% orange juice – 1 cup

Lunch

- Diet soda
- Salad made up of a one-half cup of cherry tomatoes, two ounces of albacore tuna (packed in water, two cups of field greens, and two tablespoons of balsamic vinegar as a dressing.

Dinner

- White wine – 1 Small glass
- Baked sweet potato – 1
- 3-ounce pork chop – 1
- Asparagus (steamed) – 1 cup
- Olive oil – 1 tablespoon

Snacks

- Lots of water with lemon or lime slices
- Pita bread – 1 small, and two tablespoons of hummus – 2 tablespoons

- Low-fat, sugar-free fruit-flavored yogurt – 1 serving
- One pear
- Baby carrots – 2/3 cup, with fat-free vegetable dip – 1 ounce
- Blueberries – 1 cup

Nutrition Information

- **Total Calories**: 1,218
- **Fiber**: 24 grams
- **Total Fat**: 14.6%
- **Total Carbohydrates**: 56.8%
- **Total Protein**: 22.6%
- **Sodium**: 1,615 milligrams
- **Cholesterol**: 116 milligrams
- **Sugar**: 86 grams
- **Saturated Fat**: 5.0 grams

1,500-Calorie Diet Meal Plan

To achieve a calorie intake of 1,500 every day, your DRI should have the following:

Note: DRI stands for Dietary Reference Intake

- **Fiber:** between 28 - 33.6 grams
- **Total Carbohydrates:** 130 grams
- **Total fat:** between 33 - 58 grams
- **Sodium:** 2,300 mg
- **Total Protein:** between 46 - 56 grams
- **Cholesterol:** Maximum of 200 – 300 grams
- **Sugar:** Maximum of 20 to 36 grams
- **Saturated Fat:** Maximum of 15 grams

Based on the parameters above, your menu would slightly vary depending on if you are watching your sugar intake or not. Below, you would see sample menus to guide you in creating yours.

Menu 1

Breakfast

- Whole-grain toast – 1 slice, with almond butter – 1 tablespoon
- Orange – 1
- Hardboiled egg – 1

- Plain coffee or tea – 1 cup

Lunch

- Sliced of carrots – ½ cup
- Whole-grain bread – 2 slices, Swiss cheese – 1 slice, Roast beef – two-ounce sliced, and mustard – 1 tablespoon
- Nonfat milk as a beverage – 1 cup

Dinner

- White wine – 1 small glass
- Chicken breast fillet – 1 3-ounce, with Salsa – 2 tablespoons
- Cooked black beans – ½ cup
- Cooked broccoli with lemon juice – 1 cup
- Whole-wheat dinner roll – 1, with butter – 1 teaspoon

Snacks

- Lots of water
- One nectarine – 1

- Blueberries ½ cup
- Sweetened grapefruit juice – 1 cup
- Plain yogurt – ¾ cup, with honey – 1 tablespoon
- Pecan halves – 10

Nutrition Information

- **Total Calories:** 1,498
- **Fiber:** 32 grams
- **Total Fat:** 20.5% (35 grams)
- **Total Carbohydrates:** 51.7% (201 grams)
- **Total Protein:** 23% (89 grams)
- **Sodium:** 1,934 milligrams
- **Cholesterol:** 295 mg
- **Sugar:** 87 grams
- **Saturated Fat:** 6 grams

Menu 2

This particular menu is for people that need to watch their intake of sugar, like people with prediabetes and diabetes. Rather than using sugar, you can make use of non-nutritive sweeteners.

Breakfast

- Cooked oatmeal – 1 cup, with walnuts – ½ ounces
- Grapefruit – ½
- Nonfat milk – 1 cup
- Stevia sweetener or sucralose – 1 or 2 packets

Lunch

- Baked salmon (no oil) – 3 ounces
- A salad with spinach – 1 cup, cherry tomatoes – ½ cup, feta – 1 ounce, and balsamic vinegar (no oil) – 2 tablespoons
- Diet soda – 1

Dinner

- Peeled shrimp - 6-ounces, add diced green pepper – 1 small size, sautéed in a tablespoon of garlic and olive oil
- 100% whole-grain dinner roll – 1 small
- Cooked brown rice – 1 cup
- Water with a slice of lime or lemon

Snacks

- Apple – 1
- Air-popped popcorn (butter-less) – 2 cups
- One serving sugar-free, low-fat, fruit-flavored yogurt
- Raw baby carrots – 2/3 cup, with one ounce of fat-free dip
- Strawberries – 1 cup
- Lots of water with slices of lime or lemon

Nutrition Information

- **Total Calories:** 1,496
- **Fiber:** 25 grams
- **Total Fat:** 22.4% (37 grams)
- **Total Carbohydrates:** 51.3% (193 grams)
- **Total Protein:** 26.4% (99 grams)
- **Sodium:** 1,496 mg
- **Cholesterol:** 428 milligrams
- **Sugar:** 49 grams
- **Saturated Fat:** 11 grams

1,700-Calorie Diet Meal Plan

A 1,701 Calorie Menu Without Non-Nutritive Sweeteners

Breakfast

- Eggs scrambled - 2
- 100% fruit spread – 1 tablespoon
- 100% whole-grain toast – 1 slice
- 100% apple juice as a beverage – 1 cup

Lunch

- Non-fat milk as a beverage – 1 cup
- Wrap three tomato slices, one-half cup chopped chicken, lots of lettuce, one tablespoon light mayonnaise, and 1-ounce of shredded light cheese in one whole grain tortilla.

Dinner

- One three-ounce sirloin steak
- Baked sweet potato – 1 medium size

- Cooked green beans – 1 cup
- Red wine as a beverage – 1 small glass

Snacks

- Lots of water
- One cup of 100% grapefruit juice – 1 cup
- Raw carrots – ½ cup
- Three-fourths cup plain yogurt with one tablespoon honey
- 14 walnut halves

Nutrition Information

- **Total Calories:** 1,701
- **Fiber:** 26 grams
- **Total Fat:** 29.6% (58 grams)
- **Total Carbohydrates:** 41.8% (183 grams)
- **Total Protein:** 24.3% (106 grams)
- **Sodium:** 1,326 milligrams
- **Cholesterol:** 551 milligrams
- **Sugar:** 118 grams
- **Saturated Fat:** 13 grams

A 1,705 Calorie Menu Without Non-Nutritive Sweeteners

Breakfast

- Non-fat milk – 1 cup
- 100% whole-grain toast – 1 slice, with peanut butter – 1 tablespoon
- Grapefruit – ½
- Stevia sweetener or sucralose - One packet

Lunch

- 100% whole grain dinner roll – 1 small
- Salad made with cucumber – 6 slices, mixed greens – 2 cups, cherry tomatoes- ½ cup, artichoke hearts – ½ can, cooked shrimp – 3 ounces, and balsamic vinegar for dressing – 2 tablespoons
- Diet soda

Dinner

- Black beans – ½ cup

- One burrito made with salsa – 3 tablespoons, cooked chopped chicken – ½ cup, fat-free sour cream – 1 tablespoon, low-fat shredded cheddar cheese- 1 ounce, and lettuce
- Brown rice – ½ cup
- White wine – 1 small glass

Snacks

- Raw carrots – ½ cup
- Air-popped popcorn (butter-less) – 2 cups
- One apple with ten almonds
- One orange
- Low-fat, sugar-free fruit-flavored yogurt – 1 serving
- Lots of water with slices of lemon or lime

Nutrition Information

- **Total Calories:** 1,705
- **Fiber:** 39 grams
- **Total Fat:** 19.6% (37 grams)
- **Total Carbohydrates:** 53.3% (227 grams)

- **Total Protein:** 22.7% (97 grams)
- **Sodium:** 1,717 milligrams
- **Cholesterol:** 260 milligrams
- **Sugar:** 78 grams
- **Saturated Fat:** 9 grams

Reaching Your Weight Loss Goal

After you have inputted all the required details into the weight loss calculator, the calculator would present you with a daily calorie goal. This goal contains the required number of calories you need to consume daily to be able to get to your weight loss goal within the timeframe you selected. For weight loss purposes, you would get a calorie deficit factored into the final number while calorie surplus is included in the final number for weight gain.

Calorie deficit has to do with a shortfall in energy. Whenever there is a calorie deficit, your body does not have access to the fuel that it needs to function. So, it makes use of fats stored in the body (excess weight) for fuel. Whenever you eat fewer calories than your body needs to function or burn more calories via physical activity, you create a calorie deficit. You can combine both exercise and diet to cause a calorie deficit in the body. While cutting down on your calories would help you lose weight faster, remember that it is not advisable and safe to go too low on calories. Let me explain with an example. Say, for instance, you do not exercise regularly and the weight loss calculator has advised that you would need to consume 1,200 calories daily to meet your weight loss goal and you know that you may not be able to cut down as much food as is needed to reach this number. That's not a problem as you can also include exercises to your weekly routine to lose some more calories. I have listed below some ways that this can work for you using the 1,200 calories per day need:

- If you consume 1,500 calories every day, this is 300 calories more than your advised target. You can then include 45 minutes of moderate to vigorous exercises to your daily routine to help burn the remaining 2,100 calories every week.

- If you consume 1,400 calories every day, this is 200 calories more than your advised target. You can include a HIIT workout to your schedule twice in a weekthe along with 30 minutes walks three times in a week to burn the remaining 1,400 calories per week.
- If you consume 1,300 calories every day, this is 100 calories more than your advised target. Include a short evening walk to your daily schedule to burn the remaining 700 calories every week.

In each of the scenarios that I sighted above, you went past your advised daily calorie intake but you burned them by exercising which would help you to maintain the advised calorie deficit needed for weight loss. To lose weight faster, simply add exercises to your daily routine without increasing your daily calorie intake.

Explaining High-Intensity Interval Training (HIIT),

Several people think that cardio training is just to take long but boring jogs on the treadmill or even pedaling an upright bike for an extended time. However, cardio training is all about high-intensity interval training (HIIT), which interchanges between the very high-intensity exercise rounds and either a complete rest or a low-intensity round of exercise. This is different from the 30 to 60 minutes of ongoing steady-state cardio that the majority do on the cardio machines. HIIT workouts are done in lesser time than the old cardio workout but achieve the same if not better results. Benefits of doing the HIIT workouts are:

- It raises your metabolic rate to help burn extra calories while exercising and resting.
- It increases the anaerobic and aerobic pathways that help to utilize and take in more oxygen during steady-state training. It also helps you carry out the anaerobic exercises for a longer time.
- It helps you to break through training tables.

- Increase in EPOC (excess post-exercise oxygen consumption) which leads to a longer and higher burning of calories even after you have stopped the exercise.

You can do the HIIT workouts on any cardio machine that is able to vary speed or resistance. With treadmills, you are able to grow your speed and incline while with the bike you are able to grow your speed and resistance. The elliptical trainer, on the other hand, has additional features that you can use to increase speed, resistance and ramp height. If you can get the elliptical trainer that comes with arm handles, you would be able to include the upper body in the challenge. If you are able to finish a minimum of 30 minutes cardiovascular activity of low to moderate speed on any cardio machines, then you are set to HIIT workouts using the elliptical way.

Warm-Up:

The first 5 minutes you spend on the elliptical trainer should concentrate on getting your body ready for the workout. Use 5 minutes to pedal from a low to a moderate pace just to increase body temperature as well as get the body ready for more serious work. Spend another 3 minutes playing around with increasing the machine's resistance level, speed, ramp height or even a combination of all these features to discover your maximum best.

Workout:

The workout involves alternating rounds of low and high intensities for the advised period. The intense short work phase should be the highest level that you are able to go. While on the longer, low-intensity recovery phase, lower the resistance, speed and ramp height to a pace that is okay for you to recover your breath.

Workout #1: For Beginner HIIT

Duration: 23 minutes

Warm-up
5 minutes low to moderate intensity

3 minutes to explore speed, resistance level, and ramp height to find your maximum best	
Work	Rest
30 secs	2 minutes
30 secs	2 minutes
30 secs	1:30 minutes
30 secs	1 minute
30 secs	1:30 minutes
30 secs	2 minutes
30 secs	2 minutes
Cooldown 3 minutes	

As you improve your fitness level and are able to get back faster than the suggested time, then you can reduce the time you spend resting.

Workout #2: Intermediate HIIT

Duration: 20 minutes

Warm-up

5 minutes moderate intensity to explore speed, resistance level, and ramp height to find your maximum best

Work	Rest
30 secs	1:30 minutes
30 secs	1:15 minutes
30 secs	1:00 minute
30 secs	1 minute
30 secs	45 seconds
30 secs	45 seconds
30 secs	1 minute
30 secs	1 minute

30 secs	1:30 minutes
30 secs	
Cooldown 3 minutes	

Cool down:

Reduce the speed, resistance level, and ramp height a little below the low-intensity settings. Concentrate on reducing the heart rate as well as slowing down your breath before you leave the machine.

Weight Training

Your focus during weight training sessions should be to maintain or build lean muscle mass, loss some body fat and as well increase metabolism. When you develop more active muscle tissue, it helps to increase the resting metabolic rate which would encourage your body to use up the stored-up fats for fuel.

Recommendations for Weight Training

- Carry out circuit training with minimal rest time between each set.
- Concentrate on the large muscle groups (e.g. back and legs) and high repetitions (15 reps)
- Compound exercises

Circuit Training Workout Guide

Exercise	Time
Squat with overhead press	Workout for 50 sec
Rest	Rest for 10 sec
Stationary lunge with lateral raise (right leg front)	Workout for 50 sec
Rest	Rest for 10 sec
Stationary lunge with lateral raise (left leg front holding	Workout for 50 sec

dumbbells)	
Rest	Rest for 10 sec
Plié squat/upright row (kettlebell or dumbbells)	Workout for 50 sec
Rest	Rest for 10 sec
Push-ups using a single leg knee to drive	Workout for 50 sec
Rest	Rest for 10 sec
Plank with triceps extension (dumbbells)	Workout for 50 sec
Rest	Rest for 10 sec
Alternate step-ups with hammer curls (dumbbells)	Workout for 50 sec
Repeat three times	

Other Factors to Consider

- Reduce how much time you spend watching TV.
- Reduce your sleep time, rise up early.
- Get another person involved in your workouts, a partner, a hired training, or enter a competition

When you are consistent and diligent with your exercise and eating habits, it would help a great deal in your weight loss goal.

Intermittent Fasting

In recent times, this intermittent fasting approach has gained more popularity among several dieters. One version of the intermittent fasting advises that you do not consume any food for 16 hours of the day and to take all your food intake within an 8-hour timeframe. Let me explain what this means with an example. So, if you go for this approach, you would need to eat all your food between the hours of 11 am to 7 p.m., without taking any other food between the time. We have other versions of the intermittent fasting approach. There is the 5:2 diet approach that preaches you eating all your normal food for 5 days of the week then restricts the remaining two days in the week to eating foods with about 500 to 600 calories. Another version talks about fasting for 24 hours one or two days a week.

How Effective is Intermittent Fasting for Weight Loss?

Researches have confirmed that the intermittent fast procedure could be helpful for people who want to lose weight and reduce blood sugar levels. Some dieticians have preached that rather than go for the reduced calories diet, you may go for the intermittent fast to achieve the same results. For example, one study done in June 2018 by the Journal of Nutrition and Healthy Aging advises that when you limit your food intake to an 8-hour window, you would achieve a mild caloric restriction and weight loss, without the need to count calories. It also has the added benefit of reducing your blood pressure. However, Dr. Jessica Bartfiled, an obesity medicine specialist, while agreeing that the approach could be effective, also advised that it is not for everyone. Always consult your health practitioner before you make any diet change.

Conclusion

The low-calorie diet is a broad term that covers different types and does not restrict your intake of any particular food. When you take in fewer calories, you burn excess fat faster but this diet requires careful planning and dedication. Before you start this diet, ensure to talk to your doctor or nutritionist as this would help to increase your chances of succeeding in this diet.

Other Books by Nancy Peterson

- PREDIABETES ACTION PLAN AND COOKBOOK: Your Complete Guide to Reverse Prediabetes https://amzn.to/2YnAET0
- CELERY JUICE: The Natural Medicine for Healing Your Body and Weight Loss https://amzn.to/2xTTC4Z
- ENDOMORPH DIET PLAN: The Complete Guide to Loss that Excess Fat and Stay Healthy with Paleo Diet, Exercises and Trainings Perfect for Your Body Type. https://amzn.to/2xNU3NW
- The Diverticulitis Guide to Live Pain Free https://amzn.to/2JIdixY
- Apple Cider Vinegar: Your Complete Guide on How to Use https://amzn.to/2On99VX
- Cannabis cookbook https://amzn.to/2Ztq6Cfn
- Herbal medicines https://amzn.to/2Zjcevg
- Alkaline plant-based diet for beginners https://amzn.to/33ZVNTf

Printed in Great Britain
by Amazon